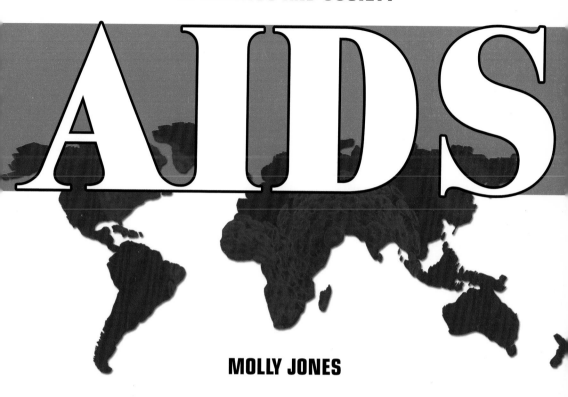

AIDS

MOLLY JONES

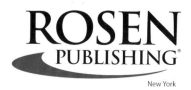

ROSEN
PUBLISHING®

New York

Published in 2011 by The Rosen Publishing Group, Inc.
29 East 21st Street, New York, NY 10010

First Edition

Library of Congress Cataloging-in-Publication Data

Jones, Molly, 1933–
AIDS / Molly Jones.—1st ed.
    p. cm.—(Epidemics and society)
Includes bibliographical references and index.
ISBN 978-1-4358-9434-1 (lib. bdg.)
1. AIDS (Disease)—Popular works. I. Title.
RC606.64.J66 2010
616.97'92—dc22

                                                             2009040246

Manufactured in the United States of America

CPSIA Compliance Information: Batch #S10YA: For further information, contact Rosen Publishing, New York, New York, at 1-800-237-9932.

On the cover: A group of human immunodeficiency virus (HIV) particles, like this one, causes severe immune system damage in human beings.

CONTENTS

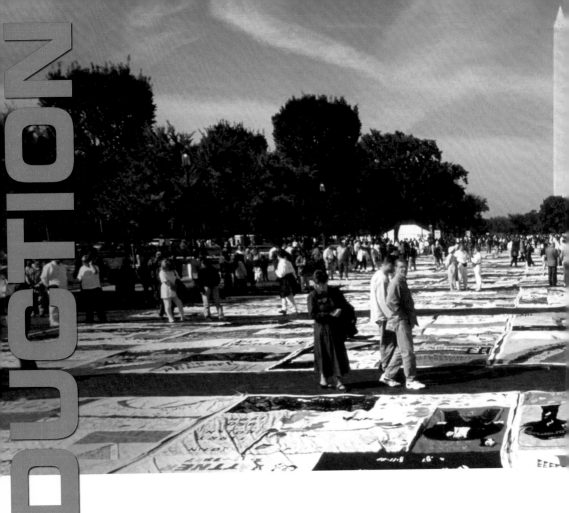

The history of acquired immunodeficiency syndrome (AIDS) and its underlying cause, infection with human immunodeficiency virus (HIV), is not one story, but many. Every victim of AIDS has different health problems, personal struggles, and losses. In the early 1980s, when the first AIDS cases attracted the attention of doctors and scientists, no treatment was known. Victims who wrote about their lives described growing more and more seriously ill, watching sick friends die, and waiting to die themselves. As research moved ahead and the cause of HIV/AIDS was finally understood, medicines were developed that delayed disability, prolonged

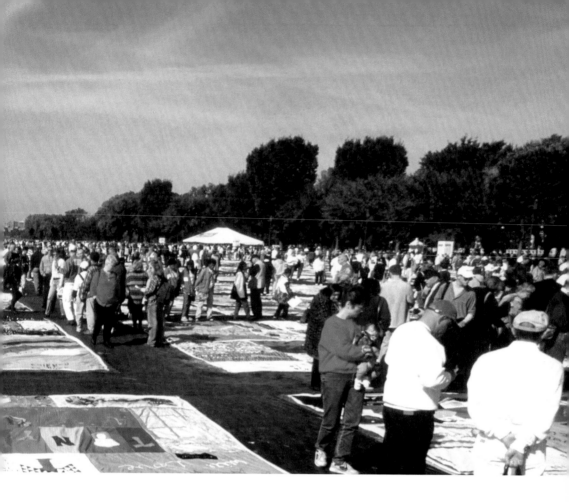

Onlookers view the AIDS Memorial Quilt displayed in Washington, D.C., in 1996. Begun in 1987, the quilt contains more than forty-four thousand panels memorializing those who have died of AIDS.

life, and decreased the spread of HIV. A positive diagnosis no longer meant death within two years but a slower journey through the disease. However, this journey often came with increasing ill health and disability and devastating medical and drug expenses. Almost three decades after the first AIDS cases baffled the medical community, no cure or preventive vaccine has been developed.

With its cause and method of spreading now understood, HIV/AIDS is a preventable disease. Yet it still runs rampant in many parts of the world and remains a major health threat even in the United States. In addition to disrupting the lives of its millions of victims, AIDS has upset the lives of whole families, communities, and entire countries. The epidemic brought confusion to politics and governments and quickly became both a national and a worldwide problem.

Although the history of AIDS is filled with illness, pain, loss, and death, it is also filled with caring, determination, and hard work. Many dedicated health researchers have spent almost thirty years working to understand the cause of AIDS, develop treatments for its victims, and find ways to prevent and cure the disease. Though AIDS has not yet been eliminated, these efforts have finally given the world hope for the future.

CHAPTER ONE

A MYSTERIOUS NEW DISEASE

Throughout human history, infectious diseases have swept through populations, sickening and killing many. Polio, Ebola, smallpox, cholera, and influenza are examples of such diseases. By the 1960s, vaccines, antibiotics, and other medicines had brought many infectious diseases under control. Smallpox had been completely eliminated and was no longer a concern. Vaccines were available to prevent polio and several other viral diseases.

No wonder, then, that in the early 1980s scientists and doctors were shocked when a new disease appeared—a disease unlike any the world had seen before. Although we now call the disease AIDS, it took a long time for scientists to understand the illness well enough to give it that name.

A Frightening New Disease

In 1981, doctors at the Centers for Disease Control and Prevention (CDC) noticed a puzzling fact. In Los Angeles, five previously healthy young men became seriously ill with a rare type of pneumonia. This pneumonia had never been a

7

threat to anyone except those who already had other major health problems. Two of the young men eventually died from complications.

Two months later, more than one hundred young men had become ill. Some had the same kind of pneumonia the first five victims had. Others had a rare type of cancer that usually affected only much older men in certain parts of Africa. Some of the victims had both pneumonia and cancer and other infections as well. Half of these one hundred men died. Something big was happening.

No one knew what was causing these rare diseases to become killers of healthy young men. Victims and their doctors knew no way to stop the sickness or keep it from spreading. Some wondered if the sickness was caused by an unknown germ that made the pneumonia and cancer worse. Others thought there must be something about the victims and their behavior that had caused their sickness. Finding the answers would take years of research.

Because the earliest victims were all homosexual men, many people believed the men's sexual behavior was causing the

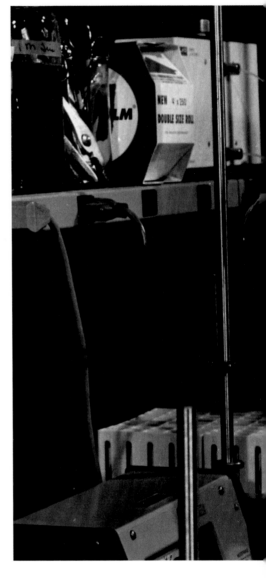

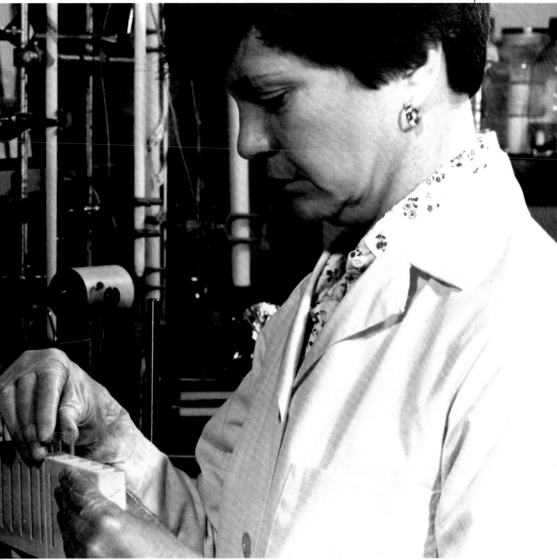

To determine the cause of AIDS, research scientists used complex technology to analyze fluid and tissue specimens from patients. At the CDC, Rosemary Ramsey applies chromatography to a specimen in 1983.

illness. In places where homophobia existed, feelings of anger and hate grew stronger toward gay men in the community.

For the victims, becoming ill with the new disease was a nightmare. Some suffered from cancerous growths. Others developed skin rashes, pneumonia, nausea, diarrhea, extreme fatigue, thrush (a painful fungal infection of the mouth), fever, brain infections, tuberculosis, ear infections, shingles (a viral disease of the nervous system), extreme weight loss, or a combination of these conditions. As the illnesses became worse, the body seemed to rot away slowly and painfully. Finally, often after years of being miserably ill, the victim would die.

False Clues and Dead Ends

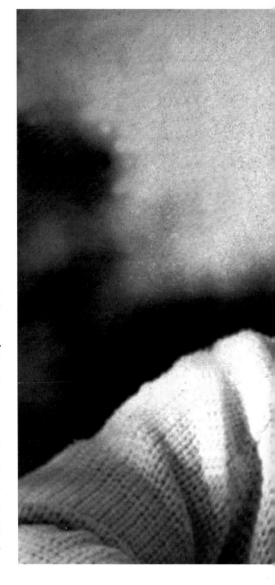

Scientists found AIDS unusual at first because it did not appear to be a single disease. Each patient would become sick with a different set of symptoms. For this reason, the condition was called a syndrome (a group of symptoms that occur together), rather than a disease.

When doctors at the CDC first began to study the victims, they found several similarities among them. First, they lived in a few large cities, such as Los Angeles, San Francisco, and New York. Second, the early victims were all young, gay men. Third, all of the victims had a very large number of sex partners. And fourth, all of the first victims had used illegal drugs.

Like false clues in a mystery story, these early observations led people to look for answers in the wrong places. Fearing that they, too, might become ill, members of the public drew incorrect conclusions from the facts. Some believed

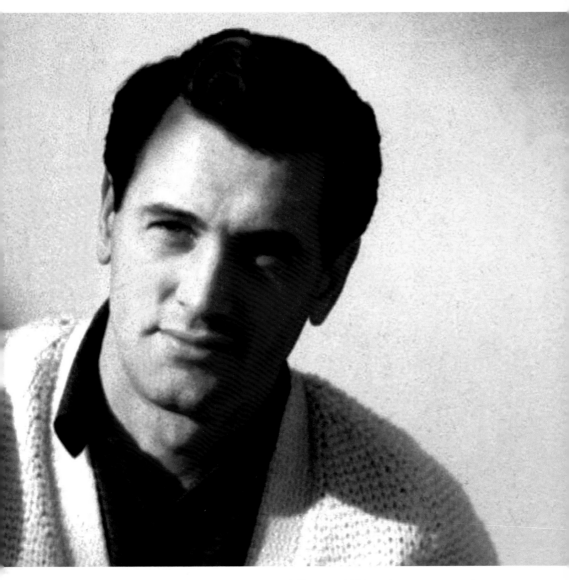

Rock Hudson, who starred in scores of films and TV series, was one of the first major Hollywood celebrities to die from an AIDS-related illness. Hudson died in 1985.

the sexual behavior of young gay men had caused their immune systems to fail. Some thought the illegal drugs were causing the illness. Still others suspected that water contamination might be spreading the illness in places where gay men gathered.

At first, many people feared they could get sick from AIDS in the same way other epidemic diseases had spread. Polio, for example, had spread from person to person through contact with an infected person or through contaminated food or drinking water. Smallpox had spread from person to person on tiny droplets of water in the air. People feared they might get AIDS by being near a person with AIDS, touching something a victim had touched, breathing air in the room a victim had entered, or drinking the local water.

When people read that the movie star Rock Hudson was a victim of AIDS, some were shocked and became even more fearful about their own risk—people felt that if a wealthy, glamorous person like Rock Hudson could get sick and die from AIDS, no one was safe. The announcement of Hudson's illness came very shortly before he died of the disease in 1985.

A Name at Last

It was 1982, more than a year after the first cases, when the strange illness was understood well enough to be given the name AIDS. By then health scientists had determined that something was attacking the body's normal ability to fight infections. The ability of the body to protect itself from disease is called immunity, which is provided by a person's immune system. When people's immune systems aren't working, they can become ill from diseases that normally wouldn't make them sick.

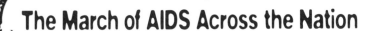

The March of AIDS Across the Nation

In June 1981, the CDC *Morbidity and Mortality Weekly Report (MMWR)* announced that five deaths were probable cases of AIDS. Two months later, in August 1981, *MMWR* reported one hundred such cases. Only one year later, in November 1982, six hundred cases were reported by the CDC. By 1994, only six years later, AIDS had become the leading cause of death for people twenty-five to forty-four years old in the United States.

In the next eight years, AIDS, now known to be associated with a virus called HIV, increased at an alarming rate. By 2002, according to the CDC Fact Sheet on HIV/AIDS, more than thirty-eight thousand people had been diagnosed with HIV/AIDS in the United States. Just four years later, in 2006, a total of more than 982,000 HIV/AIDS diagnoses had been recorded.

Once scientists understood that victims' immune systems were damaged, they knew why the disease might appear as a different set of infections in different people. They began to look for the cause of this immune system damage. Some people called the syndrome AID, or acquired immunodeficiency disease. Others called the syndrome GRID, or gay-related immunodeficiency, because they believed the syndrome was related to homosexuality.

The disease began to spread rapidly in the United States and around the globe. As women, babies, and heterosexual men began to be infected, the condition was given the name we use today, AIDS, or acquired immunodeficiency

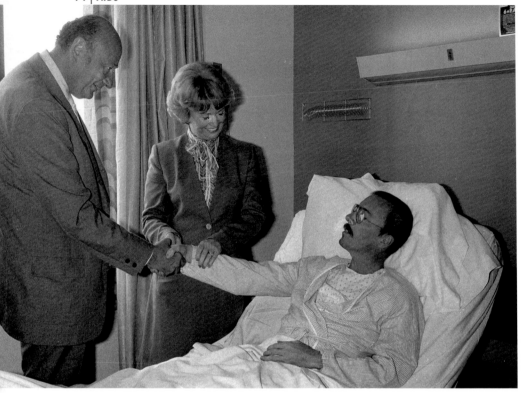

New York mayor Edward Koch and Secretary of Health and Human Services Margaret M. Heckler visit AIDS patient Peter Justice in the hospital in August 1983. Secretary Heckler promised to press Congress to double its funding for AIDS research.

syndrome. The new name recognized that anyone, not just homosexuals, could contract the disease. However, it would be some time before scientists discovered exactly what was causing victims' immune systems to fail.

CHAPTER TWO

A HISTORIC
EPIDEMIC

In the early 1980s, while researchers looked for the cause of AIDS, doctors found antibiotics helpful for treating some of the bacterial infections AIDS victims experienced, though not for treating AIDS itself. Since antibiotics are not effective against viruses, researchers suspected that a virus might be causing AIDS. Viruses were known to cause many other diseases, including some that had become worldwide epidemics. For example, polio, smallpox, Ebola, and influenza are diseases caused by viruses.

Researchers became convinced that AIDS was caused by a virus. When their studies also suggested that the virus might be contracted by contact with infected blood, some began to believe it might be spread through insect bites. Several other serious diseases were spread by insects. Malaria, for example, was spread by mosquitoes that carried the infectious organism from one person to another. Blood-feeding insects, such as head lice and bedbugs, were also suspected, but research soon ruled out insects as AIDS carriers. Many puzzles remained as scientists tried to understand this disease that seemed to have come out of nowhere.

How a New Virus Was Born

To understand how a new virus can appear, it's important to know how a virus replicates, or creates more viruses, and

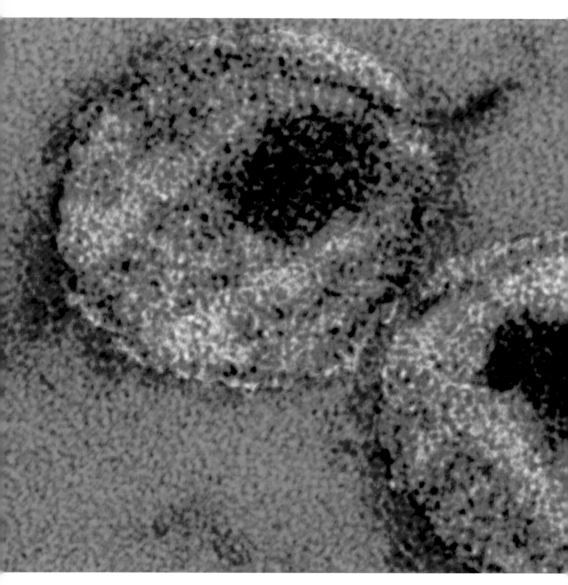

Thin sections of HIV virus particles are shown using transmission electron microscopy (TEM). Electron imaging allows examination of objects tens of thousands of times smaller than can be seen using a light microscope.

how it infects human cells. A virus is too tiny to see without a powerful microscope. Yet viruses contain genetic material, just as living organisms do. The genetic material is like a code that guides the way the organism is made and how it

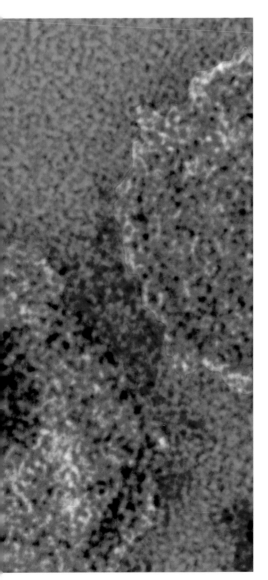

behaves. Human beings are complicated. Scientists believe human genetic material contains twenty to thirty thousand different genes.

A virus is simpler, with a smaller amount of genetic material and fewer genes. Some viruses may have fewer than ten genes, though some have many more. By itself, a virus cannot replicate and create new viruses. But when a virus infects a human cell, the virus uses parts of the human cell to replicate its genetic material, which is packaged into new viral particles.

The genetic material of a human being, which is found in every cell of the body, is made up of deoxyribonucleic acid (DNA) and ribonucleic acid (RNA). While most organisms contain both DNA and RNA, a virus contains either DNA or RNA, but not both. Viruses that have only DNA use human cells to make RNA and then DNA to produce more viruses.

Other viruses, including a type called a retrovirus, have only RNA. Once inside a human cell, a retrovirus produces DNA, which integrates its genetic code into the host cell's genetic material. The human host cell then produces RNA and proteins needed to create more retroviruses. The new retroviruses are then released to infect other cells.

Over time, accidental changes, or mutations, can take place in the DNA or RNA of an organism. These changes can be passed on to the organism's offspring. For example, the DNA or RNA of a virus that once infected only animals can mutate in a way that allows it to infect human beings.

Scientists discovered evidence that through mutation, a virus that once infected only monkeys and apes became a retrovirus. The mutated retrovirus, now called HIV, was responsible for the deadly human AIDS epidemic. Identifying that retrovirus was a big challenge to medical researchers.

Finding the Retrovirus That Causes AIDS

Scientists believe that a viral illness much like the first AIDS cases existed in Africa for many centuries, but not in human beings. Research showed that a mutation in the RNA of a monkey or ape virus had occurred about fifty years before the first Los Angeles AIDS cases were identified. That mutation produced HIV, the human immunodeficiency virus, which can infect human cells and attack the immune system. Researchers have since found records from those fifty years showing a number of strange illnesses in different parts of the world that were probably due to HIV.

As AIDS became recognized as an epidemic, many scientists looked for the cause. One leader in the search was

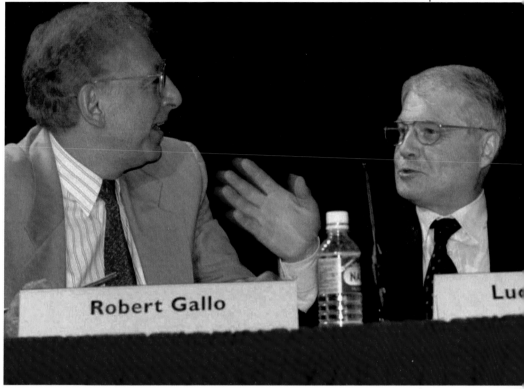

Leading AIDS researchers Dr. Robert Gallo *(left)* and Dr. Luc Montagnier *(right)* field questions at the 11th International Conference on AIDS in 1996. Many people expressed dissatisfaction with the progress made in controlling HIV/AIDS.

Dr. Robert Gallo, a scientist at the National Institutes of Health (NIH), who was the first person to identify a retrovirus in humans. Another was Dr. Luc Montagnier, a scientist with the Pasteur Institute in France, who had conducted research to describe how retroviruses replicate. Both studied cells taken from AIDS patients. In 1983, Montagnier found and named an HIV retrovirus that appeared to be connected with AIDS. In his laboratory, Gallo verified that this virus actually caused the AIDS syndrome. Montagnier was honored with the Nobel Prize for his important work, and Gallo received many other awards.

HIV: Enemy of the Immune System

By 1987, researchers had learned that HIV passed from an infected person to others through body fluids, such as blood,

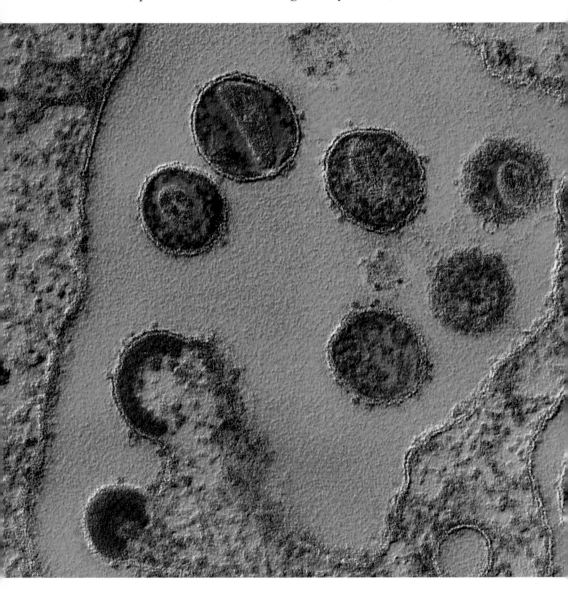

Magnified sixty thousand times by an electron microscope, HIV particles are shown budding from an infected human T cell. The spikes (green) for attaching to the host cell can be seen.

semen from male sex organs, or vaginal fluids from female sex organs. They concluded that HIV was spreading by sexual contact, blood transfusions, and shared drug needles. The infection was also spreading from pregnant women to their

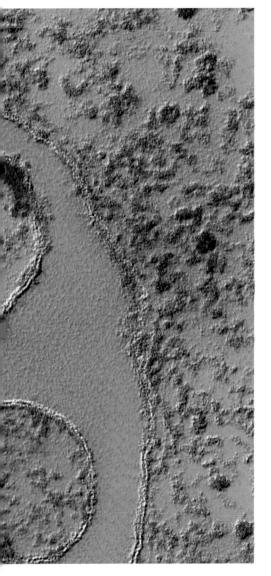

unborn children and to infants in their infected mothers' breast milk. Scientists still needed to learn how HIV caused AIDS and to find ways to prevent, treat, and cure the disease.

Human beings live with millions of microorganisms on both the inside and outside surfaces of their bodies. Bacteria, viruses, and fungi are examples of such organisms. Most of the time, these organisms don't cause problems. Sometimes, though, they rapidly increase in number, damage cells in the body, and cause illnesses.

The human body has powerful ways of defending itself against such invaders. The skin and linings on the inside surfaces of the body keep most invaders in check. When unwanted organisms do get past these surfaces, the body's immune system goes on the

attack to protect the body from infection. The reason HIV/ AIDS has been a serious problem for human beings is that it

How HIV Attacks the Immune System

The human immune system has many parts. It includes several types of white blood cells. Each type has its own defense job. Three important types of white blood cells are called granulocytes, lymphocytes, and macrophages.

Granulocytes are often able to destroy invading organisms before they can cause infection. Lymphocytes recognize and kill invading microorganisms. They are found in a body fluid called lymph that circulates throughout the body. Macrophages act like a cleanup crew, enveloping and destroying any foreign organisms that come into the body. Sometimes macrophages send signals to call other immune cells to help fight a specific infection.

Together, these three types of white blood cells protect the body from most infections. But when particular organisms manage to infect the body, special types of lymphocytes can spring into action. Among these are B cells and T cells.

When a microorganism has infected the body, B cells begin to produce antibodies, or molecules designed to attack and destroy that particular kind of organism. T cells help defend the body in several ways. One kind of T cell, the helper T cell, controls the production of antibodies by B cells. Helper T cells also control the action of both macrophages and killer T cells, which attack any foreign cells that manage to invade the body. Killer T cells also can kill host cells, including infected helper T cells.

HIV/AIDS is difficult for the immune system to fight because it can infect two of the most important immune cells, helper T cells and macrophages. The infected T cells are unable to attack the invading viruses or other organisms or to signal other immune cells to respond to invaders. The infected macrophages may actually spread the disease to other cells in the body. Weakened by HIV, the immune system is unable to fight off other diseases. Bacterial or viral infections such as pneumonia, tuberculosis, and Kaposi's sarcoma often result.

works by infecting some immune cells and bringing about the death of others, thus destroying the ability of the immune system to defend the body.

Turning the Corner at Last

Once scientists learned how HIV weakened the immune system and how the virus was spread, they could finally make progress in controlling the epidemic. Research showed that, while some viruses cause illness quickly, HIV works slowly. After HIV infects the body, months or years may pass before the person becomes sick with AIDS. A few people who are infected with HIV never develop AIDS. But even when HIV victims are not sick, they are still able to infect others. Hoping to slow the spread of HIV/AIDS, scientists eventually developed tests to determine whether or not a person was HIV positive (infected with HIV). Researchers hoped that people who knew they were infected would take steps to avoid spreading HIV to others.

Scientists also moved forward to develop drugs to treat HIV/AIDS, hoping to slow the progress of HIV/AIDS and extend the life spans of people infected with HIV.

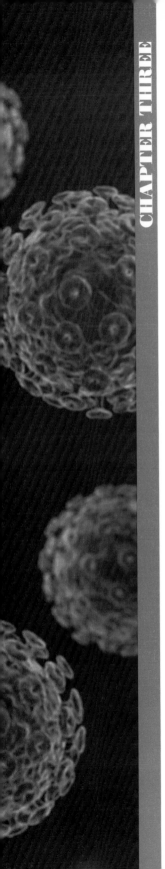

CHAPTER THREE

LIVES TORN APART

Before tests for HIV infection were developed, many victims didn't know they were infected with the virus until they began to suffer from other diseases that were complications of AIDS. The diseases that usually affected AIDS patients, such as cancer, pneumonia, and tuberculosis, were themselves major illnesses. As HIV continued to damage the immune system, a patient's diseases would grow more severe and numerous. Until effective treatments were developed, an AIDS diagnosis was a death sentence for all patients.

AIDS Before Tests or Treatments

When first infected with HIV, a person usually has no symptoms at all, though a few may have a brief period of fever, aches, swollen glands, or a rash. Most do not begin to experience AIDS-related diseases for several years after HIV infection.

As HIV replicates in the victim's cells, more and more helper T cells are destroyed. AIDS, defined by a low number of helper T cells, then sets in, and the victim has one illness after another. These illnesses are called opportunistic infections because the weakened immune system gives other infectious microorganisms the opportunity to make the patient sick. If HIV were not present, the person's immune system would usually fight

Most Frequent Opportunistic Infections

Tuberculosis (TB), a lung disease caused by bacteria, is the most common opportunistic infection worldwide. It is easy to be exposed to the TB organism and, for an HIV victim whose immune system is weakened, to become ill with it.

Pneumonia is the most common opportunistic infection in the United States and can be caused by many types of bacteria. One type of bacteria that causes many cases of pneumonia in HIV/AIDS patients is *Pneumocystis carinii*. This microorganism exists in many places in the environment, but people with healthy immune systems do not become ill from it.

Kaposi's sarcoma (KS) is a cancer caused by a virus, sometimes a herpes virus. KS usually affects the skin, mouth, nose, or eyes. When the immune system is damaged, the disease can move to major body organs and become fatal.

Other infections that occur once a person's immune system is weakened include herpes viruses of the mouth (fever blisters) and of the genital area; candidiasis (yeast infections); cancer of the lymph nodes; and other cancers. Brain damage and brain infections also occur in some HIV/AIDS patients. Near the end of life, many HIV/AIDS patients suffer from diarrhea, nausea, and weight loss.

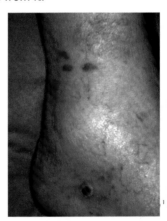

An AIDS patient's ankle and foot show skin lesions from Kaposi's sarcoma.

off such infection and prevent illness. As AIDS progresses, opportunistic infections become more numerous and severe in the patient.

The Social Scene: Accusation and Rejection

Before anyone understood the cause of HIV/AIDS or how it was spread, people feared touching HIV/AIDS patients or breathing the air they breathed. Many avoided anyone who had HIV/AIDS or was at risk for the disease. Because, as *Time* magazine reported in November 1991, gay men made up 80 percent of the earliest HIV/AIDS cases, some people tried to avoid homosexuals and stayed away from places where they might be. Some doctors and dentists did not want to treat HIV/AIDS patients for fear of coming into contact with their blood. As HIV/AIDS spread to infants and children either from their mothers or through blood transfusions, many parents

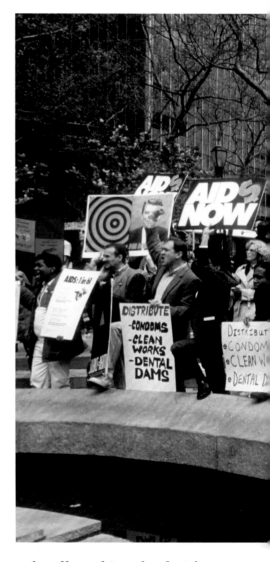

demanded that infected children not be allowed in school with their children.

Before there were accurate tests for HIV, many feared that a blood transfusion might infect them with HIV/AIDS. Once tests were developed, some wanted blood donation centers to require testing for all donors. In fact, the demand grew

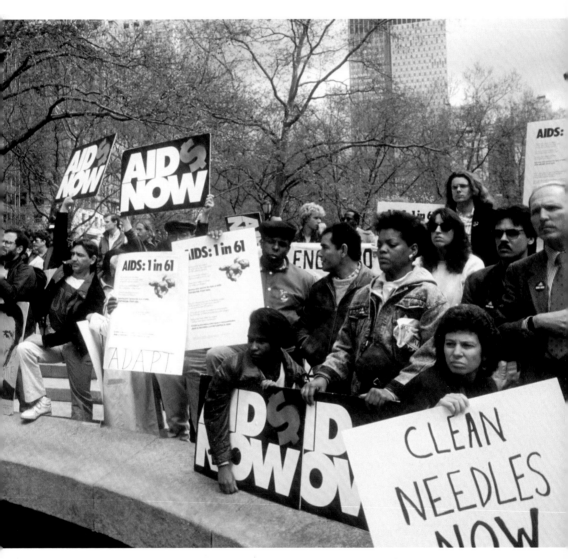

In New York and other cities, protestors demanded that the government provide clean needles, condoms, and dental dams to prevent the spread of HIV via drug injection or sexual activity.

to have everyone in the country tested. However, because of its enormous cost, such testing was never required.

Intravenous drug users slowly came to make up a larger share of the HIV/AIDS cases. Men who were infected through intravenous drug use or gay sex began to spread the infection to women through sexual contact. Women with HIV then often gave birth to infants with HIV.

Near the beginning of the epidemic, many across the country showed support for the gay population, who suffered more than any other group. They joined gay leaders in calling for more government funding to find treatments and a cure for HIV/AIDS. They also supported calls to end discrimination against homosexuals and give them the same rights other citizens had. But by the late 1980s, criticism of homosexuals and attacks on their behavior grew stronger. Religious leaders as well as political conservatives again laid blame for the HIV/AIDS epidemic on homosexuals. Some suggested that all people with HIV/AIDS be quarantined (shut away and isolated from contact with other people) so they could not spread the disease.

In 1988, a pamphlet called *Understanding AIDS* was mailed by the government to every household in the country. The pamphlet was written to explain the cause of HIV/AIDS, methods of avoiding infection, and ways to prevent the spread of the disease. Many efforts to educate people about AIDS emphasized the importance of using a condom when having sex. Condoms were considered an effective way to prevent the spread of HIV from one person to another. However, according to studies reported in the *American Journal of Public Health* in 1988 and the journal *AIDS* in 1989, a majority of the gay men surveyed didn't always use condoms during sex, even though they admitted to understanding the importance of doing so.

Medical Needs and Costs for an HIV/AIDS Victim

According to *Science* magazine in February 1988, once opportunistic infections began to show up in a person with HIV, the patient was likely to live about fifteen more months. Yet in that short time, the patient might accumulate $75,000 or more in medical bills. As the disease worsened, doctor visits, medications, and hospitalizations also increased. Many HIV/AIDS victims could not get hospital care because they had no medical insurance or because the hospitals had no space for them. As they grew too sick to work and could not pay rent or make house payments, many became homeless. Some cities provided shelters or inexpensive hotel rooms for homeless AIDS patients, but the number of patients needing care outnumbered the available spaces.

As patients became sicker, having a bed to sleep in wasn't enough. Unable to provide food for themselves, take care of their medical needs, and keep themselves and their living spaces clean, they needed assistance. To AIDS patients, it seemed the nation and government were more interested in making a moral issue of a fatal disease than in caring for victims and finding a cure.

Medicines: Successes and Failures

In 1986, the first drug that had a definite, helpful effect on patients with HIV infection was approved by the Food and Drug Administration (FDA). The drug azidothymidine (AZT) works by keeping an infected cell from producing mo[re] viruses. The hope was that, with less HIV in their cel[ls,] tims could maintain a pool of uninfected helper T c[ells]

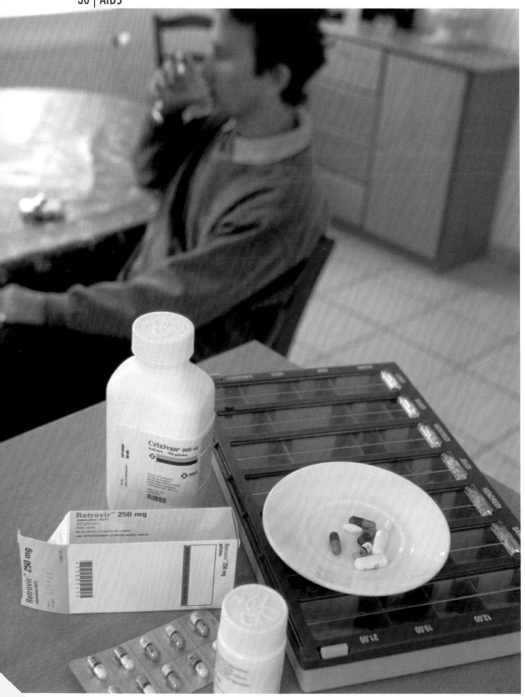

Doctors often prescribe several different drugs for HIV patients. While no drugs offer a cure, they help prevent the spread of the disease and enable patients to live longer.

thus stay healthy longer. Unfortunately, AZT was not the wonder drug everyone hoped for. A few months after a patient started taking AZT, the virus would begin to resist the drug's effect, and the patient would grow worse. A side effect of AZT was damage to the patient's bone marrow, the soft tissue inside bone cavities where new blood cells are made.

Over the next few years, other antiretroviral medications were developed that worked in different ways. The new medicines helped patients live longer and reduced their risk of spreading the virus to others. Doctors found that combination therapy (prescribing various combinations of the medicines) was more effective and caused fewer problems than using any one medication alone. However, the medications still had serious side effects that caused other health problems. Some of the side effects were nausea, diarrhea, dizziness, headache, weakness, rash, fever, and other uncomfortable conditions. Often, doctors suggested ways to help patients feel better.

Today, in addition to helping patients live longer, HIV medications greatly lower the risk that an infected mother will spread the disease to her unborn infant. In the United States and other countries where testing and medications are available, the number of infants who acquire HIV before birth has begun to decrease.

Worldwide, however, there are many areas, such as parts of Africa and Asia, where the cost of testing and medications has prevented their widespread use. In some countries governments have not made testing and medications available. In these countries, HIV/AIDS has spread widely among the people, bringing tragedy to the lives of many children and families.

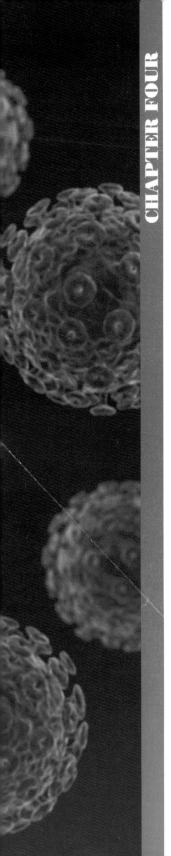

CHAPTER FOUR

THE EFFECT ON FAMILIES

Once HIV/AIDS infects a family member, the family is never the same. In addition to the medical care required by the patient, AIDS often means the sick person's responsibilities must be taken on by another family member. For example, if one parent is sick, the other parent may have to earn additional income as well as care for the children, prepare meals, and perform other household duties. If a single parent has AIDS, an older child may have to drop out of school to care for the other children, prepare meals, and care for the sick parent.

Families in Crisis

Individuals and families who live in poverty often have no health insurance. They are also more likely to become infected with HIV and to have few resources to deal with the resulting problems. Their living conditions, the difficulty of getting and using preventive measures, and their lack of access to basic health care all add to their risk. HIV/AIDS patients are more likely to be homeless than are others or to become homeless after infection. The burdens and costs of AIDS only add to the problems of those already in poverty.

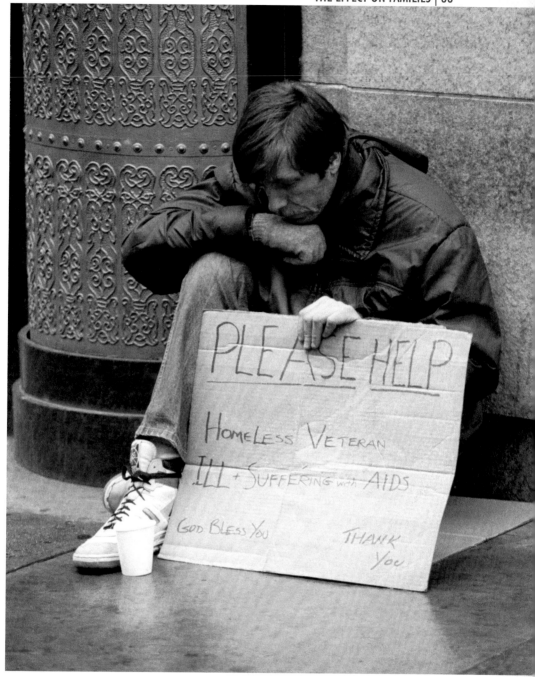

Many HIV/AIDS victims are poor when infected. Others fall into poverty when they can no longer work and face the high cost of treatment and medicines. Once their financial resources are depleted, some become homeless.

Early in the epidemic, people affected by AIDS were mostly gay men, many of whom were not married. Families were seldom affected unless they included a young male who had contracted HIV by having sex with an HIV-positive male. However, the virus can be spread in several other ways. Whenever people come in contact with the body fluids of an infected person, they risk becoming infected themselves. From 1989 and through the 1990s, more and more new infections occurred among drug users who shared needles.

Gradually, infected drug users who were heterosexual began to spread HIV/AIDS to other heterosexuals, and women began to make up a larger portion of the newly diagnosed victims. According to the 2008 CDC *HIV/AIDS Surveillance Report*, in 1985 about one in twelve new AIDS victims in the United States were women. By 2006, more than one in four new diagnoses were women. Across the globe, at least half of new diagnoses are now women.

As more and more women became infected, the disease spread to more unborn children through the mother's blood or to young infants through the mother's breast milk. Since HIV infection may not become AIDS for several years, an infection may not be diagnosed until the child is several years old or even a teenager. According to a CDC HIV/AIDS Fact Sheet, by the end of 2005, more than six thousand persons in the United States who were living with HIV/AIDS had been infected with HIV before birth, at birth, or through breastfeeding.

AIDS Among Infants and Children

In less than three decades, HIV/AIDS has created a generation of orphans. According to the Joint United Nations Programme on HIV/AIDS (UNAIDS), by 2003 more than fourteen million children around the world had been orphaned by AIDS.

AIDS and Women, the Family Caregivers

According to a national survey reported by the National Alliance for Caregiving and the AARP in 2004, 61 percent of caregivers in the United States are women. Even when a woman has health problems herself, she is often expected to care for her children, husband, and older family members. When any family member has HIV/AIDS, the woman's role as caregiver becomes more difficult. If she herself is the AIDS victim, she may not be able to get, or give herself, the care she needs. If any of her children are infected before birth or as infants, she and they will both need treatment and may be ill at times.

Because more low-income families are affected by HIV/AIDS than those with higher incomes, job loss, high medical expenses, and the cost or lack of health insurance are frequent problems. According to the *Nation's Health* in June/July 2005, Medicaid, a government health insurance program for low-income families, pays for more HIV drugs than any other source. Yet when applications for Medicaid to pay for HIV drugs increased, the government was working to cut Medicaid funds. Large numbers of children as well as infected adults had no other source for their medication. Even today, HIV-infected patients, especially women, often go without life-saving medicine in order to have money for food and a place to live for their families.

Children whose families are broken or nonexistent are at higher risk for poverty, lack of adequate food, and various kinds of abuse than children whose families remain whole.

Also in 2003, according to UNAIDS, approximately 2.5 million children under age fifteen were living with HIV/AIDS around the globe. Five hundred thousand had already died. When children are infected before birth with HIV, about one in five will become very ill in the first year of life. Most of these children will die by age four. Others may not develop serious

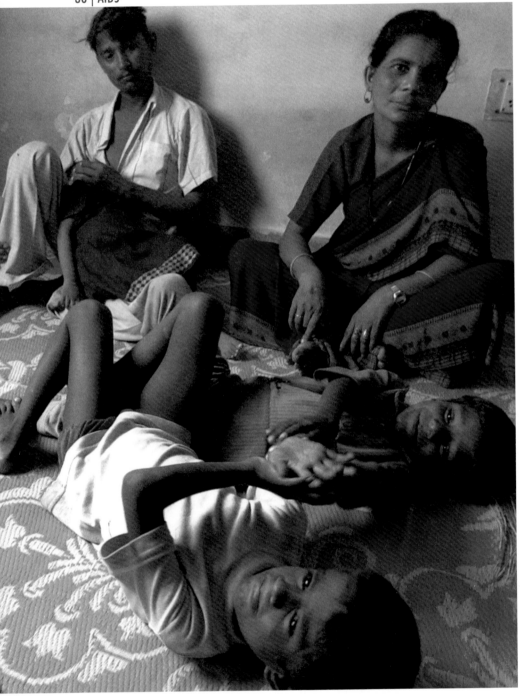

In some countries, such as India, HIV infection rates continue to rise sharply in the twenty-first century. Above, two HIV-positive children and two adults are being cared for in a shelter in New Delhi.

illnesses for several years. Many will live past age nine, and a few will still appear healthy beyond that age.

Before the cause and spread of HIV/AIDS was well understood, many parents of schoolchildren wanted infected children kept out of schools and other places children gathered. They feared their children could catch the disease through any contact with infected children. Children known to have AIDS were sometimes avoided and often faced discrimination.

The lives of children around the world are strongly affected by AIDS. AIDS has the power to impoverish children, make them homeless, prevent them from getting an education, make them into caregivers of sick parents, and take away their parents through death. Until HIV/AIDS can be prevented and cured, millions of children will never be able to live healthy, safe lives within a family.

TEN GREAT QUESTIONS
to ask a DOCTOR

1   What causes AIDS?

2   What are the symptoms of HIV and AIDS?

3   Who is at risk of getting HIV and AIDS?

4   How can I avoid getting AIDS?

5   How can I find out if I am HIV positive?

6   If I am HIV positive, what should I do?

7   Are there medicines that will cure HIV or AIDS?

8   Can I get AIDS by having a blood transfusion?

9   Should I stay away from people who have AIDS?

10   Is there a vaccination that will prevent AIDS?

CHAPTER FIVE

AIDS IN THE COMMUNITY

In its first two decades, the HIV/AIDS epidemic brought serious problems to many communities around the country. The loss of lives and health, the fear, blame, and distrust among citizens, and the shifting of community resources from other needs to the HIV/AIDS problem put a strain on community health and social services, as well as local governments. Two parts of the HIV/AIDS problem that fell heavily on communities were managing the cost of treatment and preventing the spread of the disease.

Preventing the Spread of HIV/AIDS

While the federal government could support research and provide information, the ground war on HIV/AIDS—providing medical care and preventing its spread—was a person-to-person challenge. Testing for infection, education programs, and distribution of condoms and needles had to be carried out by people and agencies within the community. Providing HIV medications to victims was a preventive strategy as well as a health program. Research showed that those

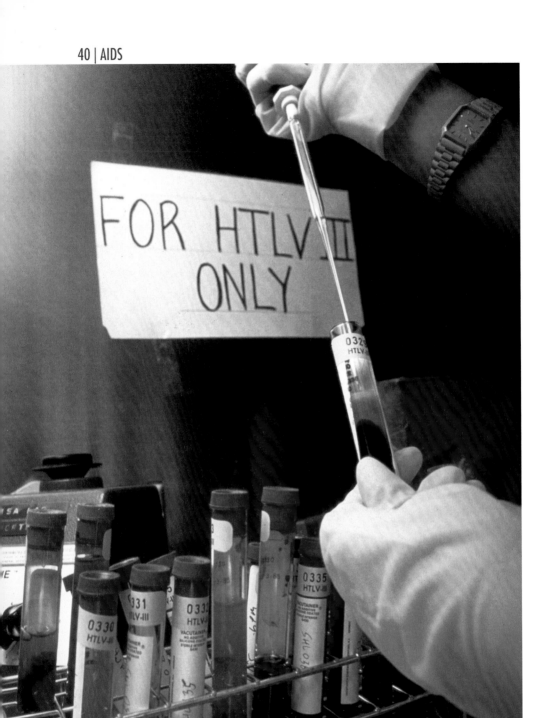

To avoid spreading HIV through blood transfusions, health department technicians test all donated blood for infection. Any blood found to contain HIV antibodies is discarded.

who took medications to reduce the virus in their systems were less likely to infect others.

The methods health agencies had used to manage other infectious diseases—sanitation, purification of drinking water, insect control, food inspection, quarantines, sewer construction—had no effect on the AIDS epidemic. Once they knew the disease was able to spread through blood transfusions, health officials worked to make sure the blood supply in local blood banks was safe. The first kits to test for HIV infection finally began to arrive at blood banks and plasma centers early in 1985.

Testing for HIV

The tests used on donated blood did not identify HIV in the blood samples. Instead, they determined if the blood contained HIV antibodies, proteins made by the body to specifically attack HIV. The presence of HIV antibodies would show that the donor's immune system was fighting HIV. If the antibodies were found in donated blood, the blood would not be used.

Testing donated blood cost much less than testing individual donors to determine if they were HIV positive. If a unit of donated blood tested positive, the blood could be discarded without being retested for accuracy. However, if a person tested positive, a second, more expensive test was needed to be sure the first result was accurate. The two tests together gave a reliable result.

Bitter arguments surrounded testing blood for HIV infection. Though blood banks promised that donors' names would be kept private, some still feared that a positive result might cost them their jobs or result in other discrimination. Today, all donated blood is tested for HIV.

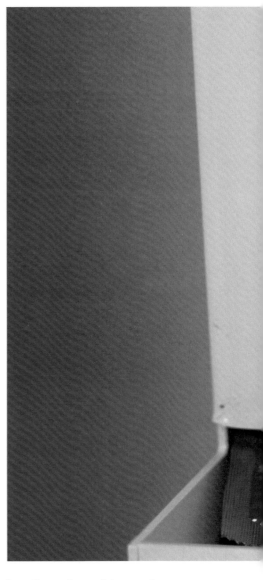

Feelings were even more divided about testing individual citizens. Some wanted everyone tested. Others thought all people considered at high risk of spreading infection should be tested. Many, though, believed that testing should be an individual choice and that the results should be private to prevent discrimination. In the end, decisions about who should be tested were left to the states, and HIV testing has remained mostly voluntary.

Being tested is the only way a person can know if he or she is HIV positive. Since the test measures whether the virus has been present long enough for the immune system to produce antibodies, a second, later test may be needed to be certain of an accurate result. Today, testing is easier than ever. A rapid test is now available that takes less than thirty minutes, and testing is free in many places.

Making Sex and Drugs Safer

The most common ways to contract HIV are by engaging in unprotected sex and by using a drug needle an infected

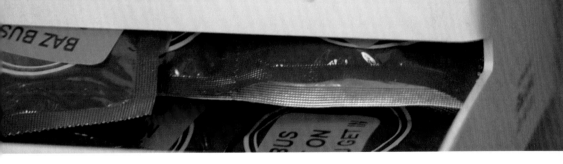

AKE A FREE
CONDOM
help fight
AIDS

To prevent the spread of HIV through sexual activity, some government and health officials advocated making free condoms available in public places. The practice aroused heated controversy.

person has used. As the AIDS epidemic developed, community health workers looked for ways to reduce the number of new cases. Some favored making free condoms available in convenient places and providing free, clean needles to drug users. Like HIV testing, these ideas were strongly favored by many people and strongly opposed by many others.

Health workers used posters, pamphlets, mailings, classes, and workshops to teach how HIV/AIDS spreads and how condoms can reduce the risk of infection. In some states, health agencies began putting free condoms in public places, including schools, where people could get them easily. Many parents reacted angrily. To them, putting condoms in schools implied that sexual activity among students was acceptable.

Similar objections were raised to the idea of providing free, clean needles to drug addicts who turned in their used needles. Community health workers whose goal was to reduce the spread of HIV/AIDS strongly favored the program. To them, the cost of providing needles seemed small compared to the cost, in money and suffering, of new victims. Those who objected believed the program supported and encouraged drug addiction. They believed the same effort and money should be used to fight drug abuse and treat drug addicts, rather than making drug use easier.

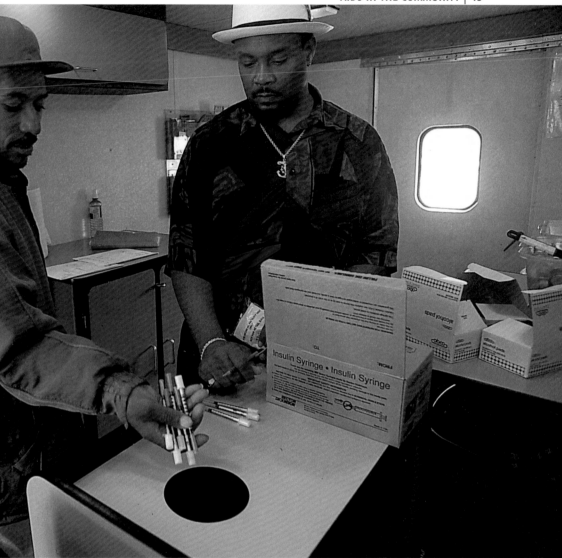

A drug addict exchanges used needles for free, clean needles. Like the practice of providing free condoms, giving free needles to addicts was strongly opposed by many people.

The challenge the disease poses to community health and social agencies has steadily increased over the three decades of the AIDS epidemic. According to a UNAIDS report in 2001 and an American Psychological Association report in 2009,

Who Should Pay the AIDS Bill?

In 1987, according to estimates in *Public Health Reports*, the medical expense for a single AIDS patient in the fifteen months of life after diagnosis was $75,000. Other financial burdens to victims and families included lost wages and child care. Once testing and drug therapy were developed, victims lived longer but had even higher medical costs.

Because of the high cost of HIV/AIDS, some insurance companies were refusing to insure those at high risk of infection, such as men suspected of being gay. This left public community hospitals to treat more and more AIDS patients who often could not pay their bills. Hospitals sometimes had to charge other patients more in order to cover the growing costs of AIDS care.

In addition to the financial costs of AIDS, local governments had to deal with an atmosphere of fear and distrust. Angry citizens blamed the lifestyle and behavior of gays for putting everyone else at risk. They claimed that the rights of homosexuals and AIDS victims were being given more importance than the rights and health of the whole population.

In the 1990s, the federal government gradually increased funding both for AIDS research and health care. By that time, communities faced several other costly challenges: testing for infection; preventing the spread of the disease through education; distributing free condoms and clean drug needles to prevent infections; and making the expensive HIV medications available to patients.

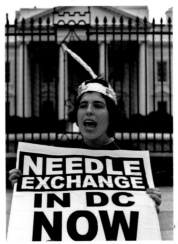

HIV/AIDS activists demand government and community help to prevent spreading HIV.

HIV/AIDS affects those with low socioeconomic status—that is, people who are poorer or less educated—at a higher rate than those of higher status. Some HIV/AIDS patients are even homeless and without any family support. While many are poor before becoming infected, many others become poor because of the unending cost of medicines, loss of income, and increased living expenses.

A single patient's medicine and care can cost tens of thousands of dollars. According to a 2005 study reported in the Raleigh *Sunday News and Observer*, taxpayers in North Carolina spent $145 million for Medicaid assistance to AIDS patients in that one year. The growing cost of HIV/AIDS has left communities and agencies with shrinking funds and resources for other important health and social needs.

Myths and Facts

MYTH HIV/AIDS can be spread by mosquito bites, drinking fountains, public toilets, or through the air an infected person has breathed.

FACT HIV/AIDS is not spread by touch, insect bites, saliva, water, or air. Neither is it spread by casual contact, such as kissing, hugging, or holding hands. HIV/AIDS is spread only by contact with the body fluids of an infected person, such as blood, fluids from male or female sex organs, or by mother's milk.

MYTH Antibiotics can cure HIV/AIDS.

FACT Antibiotics can cure some opportunistic infections caused by bacteria, but they have no effect on HIV. There is currently no cure for HIV or AIDS.

MYTH The AIDS epidemic is going away.

FACT The number of new cases continues to increase worldwide. While new cases in the United States did decline starting in 1984, they began to increase again in 2001.

MYTH Being HIV positive is not a problem when infected people take the prescribed medicine.

FACT The HIV medicines keep most infected people healthier and help them live longer. However, many of the medications have serious side effects and are very expensive. Also, as drug-resistant strains of HIV develop, the medications can become less effective.

CHAPTER SIX

GOVERNMENT ACTION

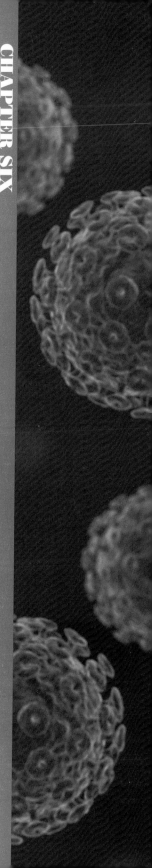

When the first five cases of AIDS appeared in 1981, health researchers in President Ronald Reagan's administration had no idea how serious the epidemic would become. In 1982, when the CDC reported almost six hundred cases, half of whom had died, the problem still seemed small compared to past epidemic diseases or major illnesses, such as heart disease, cancer, or diabetes. Government agencies put only a small fraction of their budgets into AIDS research and care.

The gay community and its supporters believed the government wasn't doing enough to find a solution or to care for victims. They claimed that if the major victims were heterosexuals, the government would be putting more funds and resources into the problem.

AIDS in the Reagan Era

Actually, by 1983, just two years after the disease was first known, the government did recognize AIDS as a major public health concern. In fact, the Public Health Service declared AIDS its number-one priority. That year, the total government budget for AIDS research and

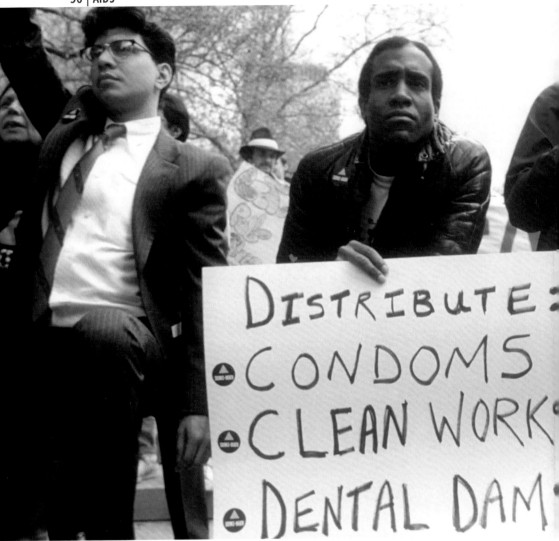

During the Reagan presidency, demonstrators protested the inadequate government response to the growing AIDS crisis. Though Reagan appointed a National Commission on AIDS, he took little action to implement its recommendations.

care was three times as much as the first year, and, by 1985, almost twenty times as much.

While some believed government wasn't doing enough for AIDS, others opposed any public spending to help communities and hospitals deal with AIDS. California congressman

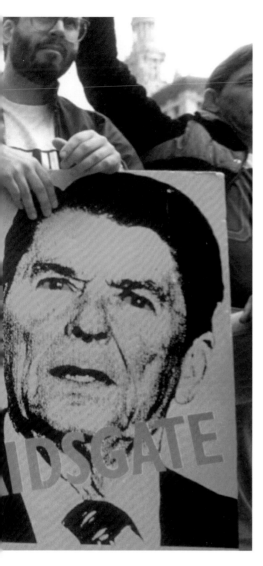

William Dannemeyer spoke for many angry citizens. In the *Los Angeles Times* in February 1986, Dannemeyer accused the homosexual community and its supporters of putting the civil rights of AIDS patients and high-risk groups ahead of the civil rights and health of the general public.

Between 1981 and 1989, the government gradually did become more involved with HIV/AIDS issues, and funding for the disease steadily increased. However, some say that President Reagan himself had little to say about HIV/AIDS and that he failed to use all the funds Congress provided.

Some in Reagan's administration thought that the situation was critical and that the government should take more action. In 1986, a report by Surgeon General C. Everett Koop supported more sex education in the schools and more public education to combat the spread of HIV/AIDS. Many citizens and members of Congress opposed Koop's ideas. They didn't want their children exposed to these topics or embarrassed by having them presented in school. They believed parents should deal with sex education in the way they saw fit.

Unfortunately, reports in 1987 and 1988 were discouraging for Koop and those who favored his plan. Many public schools had offered sex education for twenty-five years. However, studies showed little effect on the behavior of teenagers or on their views about sexual behavior. Studies also showed that educating high-risk adult groups about ways to avoid HIV/AIDS, such as using condoms, had little effect on their actual behavior. Though the reports were disappointing, government agencies continued with their education efforts. In the next few years, the efforts began to pay off as the number of new infections started to drop.

While he was president, Reagan appointed a National Commission on AIDS to advise him on AIDS concerns. The commission's first report in 1988 advised the government to protect the rights and privacy of HIV/AIDS victims and to prevent discrimination against them or high-risk groups. The commission also favored more government support for HIV/AIDS care and treatment programs and urged rapid approval of new medications to treat HIV/AIDS. While the Reagan administration did not publicly oppose the report, little was done to put the suggestions into practice.

Bush and the Politics of AIDS

During George H. W. Bush's presidency, from 1989 to 1993, the total number of HIV/AIDS cases reported by the CDC passed one hundred thousand with no preventive vaccine or cure in sight. The HIV/AIDS epidemic was now growing more serious every day.

Unlike Reagan, Bush spoke out often about HIV/AIDS. He expressed sympathy for victims and their families and supported more government activity and spending in all parts of the HIV/AIDS battle. Papers in the Bush library show that

The March of AIDS Around the Globe

According to UNAIDS, in 2001 there were twenty-nine million people living with HIV. During that year, there were 3.2 million new HIV infections, and 1.7 million people died of AIDS. By 2007, there were 33.2 million people living with HIV. During that year, there were 2.5 million new HIV infections, and 2.1 million people died of AIDS.

Around the world, two-thirds of adults and nine out of ten children who are HIV positive live in sub-Saharan Africa (the countries in Africa south of the Sahara Desert). United Nations agencies estimate that by 2004, fifteen million children under age eighteen had lost one or both parents to AIDS. From 1981 through 2007, twenty-five million people around the world died of AIDS. UNAIDS reports that AIDS is now one of the leading causes of death worldwide and the number one cause of death in Africa.

during his presidency HIV/AIDS funding increased 170 percent. By 1988, far more was being spent on HIV/AIDS research, prevention, and treatment than on any other disease, even though HIV/AIDS affected a relatively small number of people.

Many still thought Bush showed too little leadership during the HIV/AIDS crisis. Others argued that too much was being spent on HIV/AIDS programs. They cited CDC reports showing ten times as many cancer deaths each year as AIDS deaths.

Bush convinced some that he was committed to fighting AIDS when he appointed a popular basketball star, Earvin "Magic" Johnson, to the National AIDS Commission. In 1991, Johnson had announced that he was HIV positive, explaining that he had become infected through heterosexual activity.

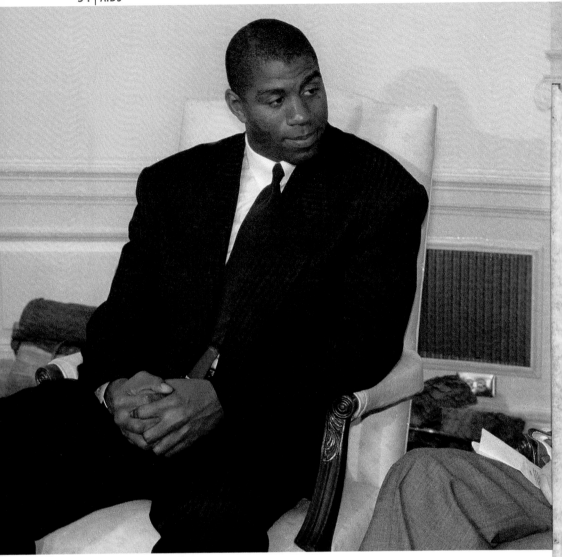

Basketball star Magic Johnson was appointed by President George H. W. Bush to the National Commission on AIDS. Johnson resigned after eight months, saying President Bush had "dropped the ball" in the fight against AIDS.

The appointment of Johnson was praised by some people. They believed that having an admired athlete talk about his own HIV infection would convince others to take HIV/AIDS more seriously. Many thought the appointment was a political

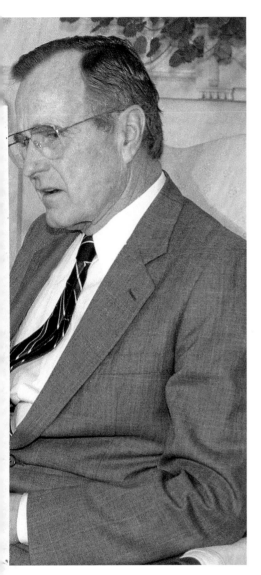

move on Bush's part. They claimed that Johnson had no qualifications that would contribute to the objectives of the commission.

The AIDS Battle Widens

Funding for the HIV/AIDS battle increased while Bill Clinton was president (1993–2001), and the government took other steps to maintain public interest and support. A White House AIDS coordinator was appointed, along with an AIDS task force to set research and treatment priorities. President Clinton also spoke out about his plan for fighting HIV/AIDS.

According to CDC estimates, after reaching a peak of about 160,000 new HIV cases per year in the mid-1980s, the number dropped to about one-fourth as many new diagnoses by the year 2000. The number of AIDS deaths also declined, dropping from a high of about fifty thousand per year to below twenty thousand by the end of the decade. The government's programs of education, research, drug development, and prevention appeared to have changed the direction of the AIDS epidemic.

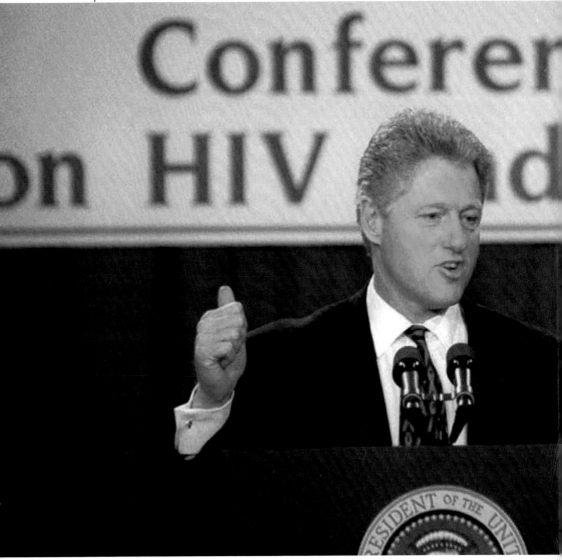

At the 1995 White House Conference on HIV and AIDS, President Bill Clinton focused national attention on the need to find both a cure for HIV and a vaccine to prevent further infections.

Worldwide, though, the situation was very different. According to estimates made by the United Nations World Health Organization (WHO), by the year 2000, fifty million people around the globe had been infected with HIV, and

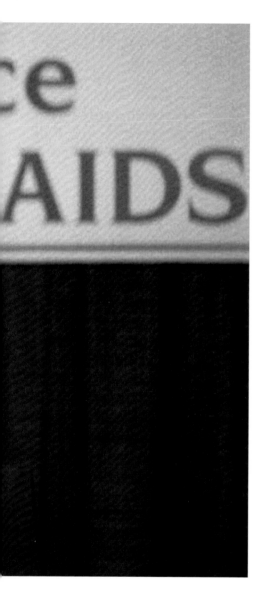

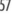

21.8 million had died of AIDS. The poorest countries in Africa were the hardest hit by the disease. There, testing and medication were far too costly for most people to afford. While the infection and death rates in the United States were beginning to level off, those in areas including Africa, India, and the Caribbean islands were rising. Other countries, the United Nations, and private groups began to offer funding and medical help. Early in his term, President George W. Bush pledged $15 billion from the United States to fight global HIV/AIDS over the next ten years.

The money was greatly needed. But, as we'll see in the next chapter, money would not stop the march of HIV/AIDS around the world.

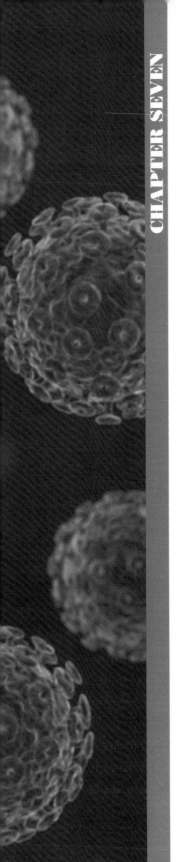

CHAPTER SEVEN

PREVENTION AND TREATMENT TODAY

In the United States, by the end of the twentieth century, HIV/AIDS no longer seemed the threat it had been before. Many now thought of AIDS as a chronic disease, a condition someone could manage for life, like diabetes or heart disease. An HIV-positive diagnosis was no longer considered a death sentence. Unfortunately, people's reactions to this news had surprising results.

A Shift into Reverse

In the 1990s, HIV infection rates and AIDS death rates had been steadily dropping, and combination drug therapy was helping patients live longer and reducing the spread of infection. For some, the lower rates showed that prevention efforts were working and should be pushed even harder. Others behaved as if getting AIDS was no longer a problem and returned to unsafe sex practices. As the new century began, infection rates were no longer falling. In 2001, according to CDC estimates, the number of AIDS cases in the United States actually rose for the first time in years.

Unsafe sexual behavior was not the only concern of those working to control HIV.

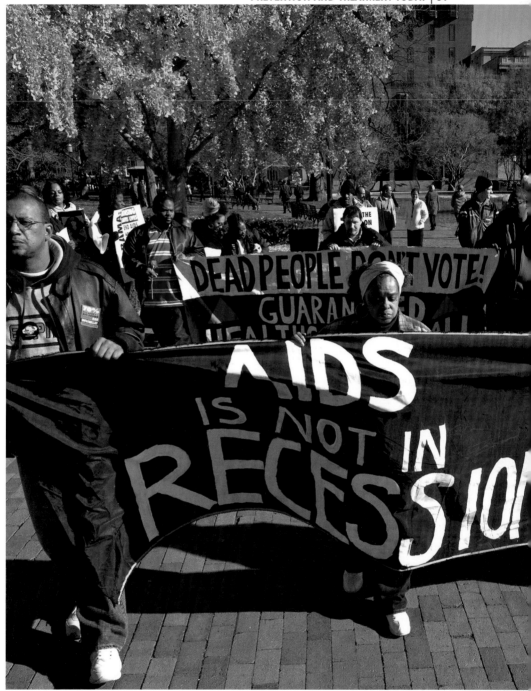

AIDS activists marched near the White House on World AIDS Day, December 1, 2009, to remind onlookers that, though the economy was in recession, AIDS remained a major threat.

Long-term use of HIV medications created problems, which sometimes discouraged patients from continuing their treatments. For the medicines to work, a patient had to take as many as thirty-two to forty pills daily, taking each drug in a certain way at a certain time of day. Often, the medicines had unpleasant side effects, such as nausea, diarrhea, fatigue, weight loss, skin rashes, or headache.

Another problem was the high cost of HIV medications. With each drug costing several thousand dollars per year, a patient's total medical costs were far higher than most could afford. Often, those who had no insurance and could not afford the medications simply did without them. Others sought government help through Medicaid. By the late 1990s, Medicaid was spending $1.3 billion per year on HIV/AIDS.

Important People in AIDS Research and Activism

From the early 1980s to today, many dedicated scientists, doctors, government officials, and citizens have worked to help the world understand and gain control of the AIDS epidemic. Below are a few of them.

Dr. Robert Gallo, an NIH scientist, and his team of researchers, discovered human retroviruses in 1976. His research helped verify that the HIV retrovirus, discovered by Dr. Luc Montagnier, was the cause of AIDS. Gallo won many awards for his outstanding work with viruses.

Dr. C. Everett Koop, surgeon general in the Reagan administration, recognized in the mid-1980s how serious the AIDS epidemic was becoming. Stressing the importance of preventing infection, Koop strongly advocated monogamy, or having sex with only one person. In spite of opposition from others in the government and across the country, he worked to promote sex education in schools and to educate the public about the importance of using condoms.

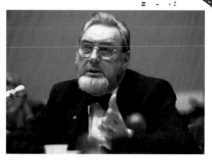

Surgeon General C. Everett Koop advocated sex education, condom use, and monogamy to curb the spread of AIDS.

Larry Kramer is a gay playwright and activist. From the earliest days of AIDS, Kramer repeatedly spoke out against the government's weak response to the disease. He also pressured the gay community to change behaviors that spread HIV/AIDS. Eventually, in 1988, Kramer himself was found to be HIV positive.

Dr. Luc Montagnier, a French scientist at the Pasteur Institute in Paris, discovered the HIV/AIDS retrovirus in 1983 while studying tissue from an AIDS patient. Montagnier received the 2008 Nobel Prize in Medicine.

Ryan White was born in 1971 with hemophilia, a blood disease that causes frequent bleeding because the blood doesn't clot properly. As a child, Ryan became infected with HIV through transfusions of blood proteins from donors, and he developed AIDS in his teen years. Many parents tried to block him from attending school with their children. But White fought against ignorance about AIDS and discrimination. He died before graduating from high school. In 1990, just before he died, Congress passed the Ryan White CARE Act to assist HIV/AIDS victims.

Dr. David Ho, a research scientist, discovered an important fact about HIV that greatly improved treatment for victims. Because HIV does not make a victim sick for several years, many believed the virus was inactive during that period and that treatment would not be effective. Ho did not believe that theory. He proved that the virus began to multiply immediately after infection and that treatment should begin as soon as HIV is diagnosed.

Like many drugs, HIV/AIDS medicines can become less effective over time. When drugs fail to destroy all of the viruses in a patient's system, due to missed doses or to mutation of the virus, those remaining are the ones most able to resist the drugs. The offspring of these resistant viruses also tend to be resistant to the drugs. Over time, the patient's body will contain more and more drug-resistant viruses, and the drugs will be less effective. Also, if the patient infects another person, the new patient will be infected with a resistant strain of the virus.

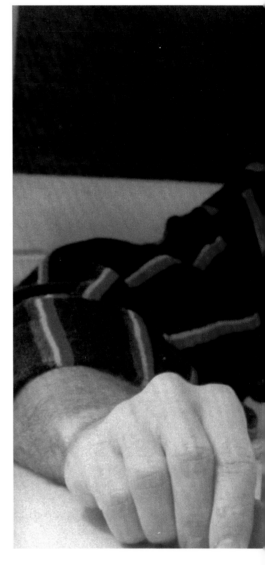

HIV is especially good at mutating to produce resistant viral strains. By 2001, the CDC estimated that more than half of patients were infected with resistant strains of HIV.

Living with HIV/AIDS

As improved drugs have become available, many younger, unin-fected members of high-risk groups see no reason to fear HIV, and some take unneces-sary risks. But others, who have watched friends and family members suffer and die from AIDS, take a different view.

Patients who have lived for years with HIV infection and treatment also see AIDS differently. No matter how much better the medicines are than in earlier years, life with AIDS is still difficult, unpleasant, and costly.

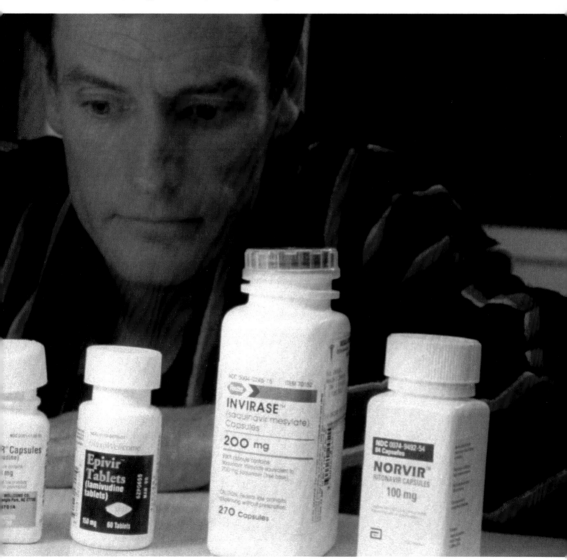

Dr. Mahlon Johnson, above, was infected with HIV while performing an autopsy on a person who died of an AIDS-related illness. Here, he takes his daily dose of HIV medications.

In January 2008, the *New York Times* interviewed patients who had been on HIV/AIDS drug therapy for ten to twenty years. The *New York Times* also interviewed doctors who cared for these longtime patients. Almost all of the patients suffered from serious conditions, such as illnesses of the liver, heart, blood, brain, kidneys, and bones. Their doctors reported that, although the patients were only middle-aged, they had diseases and disabilities usually seen only in much older people. Combination therapy has only been used for a short time. It will take many more years for researchers to know for certain what the long-term effects of HIV/AIDS therapy are likely to be.

A Look Over the Horizon

Medical research has successfully controlled many epidemic diseases in the past. Smallpox, for example, has now been eliminated, and polio has now been controlled in parts of the world by an effective vaccine. Huge challenges remain, though, before research can claim victory over the HIV/AIDS epidemic. Though medication therapy has changed the outlook for HIV/AIDS victims in the United States, neither medication nor prevention methods have been completely successful.

Serious difficulties exist in developing a preventive vaccine for HIV, as well as a vaccine for those already infected with HIV. As with many diseases, the body's immune system fights HIV by making antibodies designed to destroy the virus. However, once a person is infected with HIV, the immune system becomes less able to produce antibodies to control the virus. The amount of virus in the body gradually increases until the available antibodies can no longer control the disease. Since vaccines often work by causing the immune system to produce antibodies, HIV's ability to stop the production of antibodies can prevent a vaccine from working.

Another problem is HIV's ability to mutate and produce viruses that are resistant to both antibodies and drugs. An antiretroviral drug or a vaccine may be effective at first, but once the virus evolves, the vaccine or the medicine may no longer work. Currently, research scientists are working to overcome these problems.

The Global Challenge

According to UNAIDS estimates, the number of people living with HIV around the world has risen from fewer than ten million in 1990 to more than thirty-three million in 2007. Facts presented in UNAIDS studies show an urgent need to bring public attention back to the HIV/AIDS epidemic. First, most people who are HIV positive have not been tested and don't know they are infected. Second, fewer than one in five people at risk around the world know about and have ways of preventing HIV infection.

Since women make up nearly half of those living with HIV, lack of preventive methods puts their future children at greater risk. Also, worldwide, fewer than one in ten infected pregnant women receive treatment drugs. As a result, they risk infecting their infants. In fact, each day fifteen hundred children around the globe are newly infected with HIV, and most are newborns infected before birth.

Until a cure and a vaccine are found, it is urgent that ways are developed to improve the outlook for millions in other parts of the world. While HIV prevention and medication remain less than perfect in the United States, even bigger problems exist in less developed countries. Prevention methods and medication are not as available in those countries. Lack of education, poverty, the low status of women, and the failure of some governments to support efforts to prevent and treat HIV/AIDS also contribute to the problem.

The United States and other countries in the developed world have begun to give generous amounts of money and assistance to help poorer countries fight the epidemic. Also, some drug companies have greatly lowered the cost of HIV

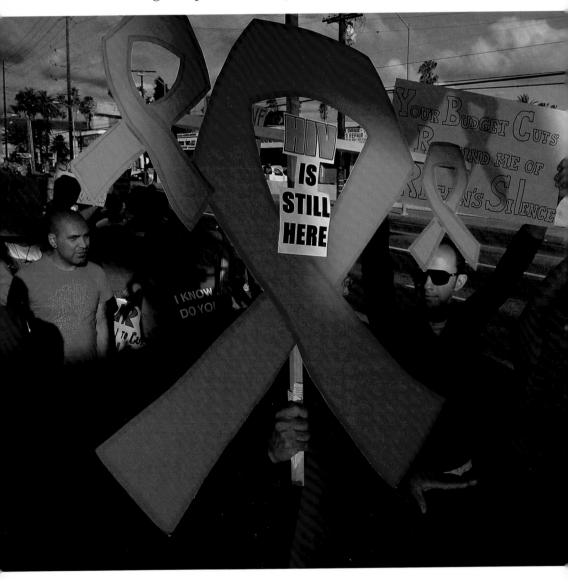

Many states were forced to make sharp budget cuts in 2009. AIDS patients in California, shown above, and other states demonstrated to protest the decreases in funding for AIDS services.

medications in undeveloped countries so more people can be treated. But even the lower prices are still beyond what most people infected with HIV can afford.

HIV/AIDS thrives in places where people are poor and

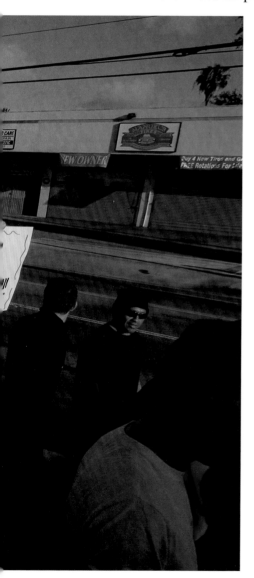

uneducated. New strategies are needed to help people understand HIV/AIDS, learn how to prevent infection, and successfully treat the disease. Strategies to reduce poverty and raise education levels in poor regions are essential to improve the health of both the people at risk for infection and those who are already infected. Also, since women in many parts of the globe have little control over their bodies and sex lives, helping them receive an education and obtain personal rights is essential if HIV/AIDS is to be controlled.

While government leaders in all countries have great responsibility for the global fight against HIV/AIDS, citizens can help by insisting that their governments expand efforts to control the worst epidemic the world has ever faced.

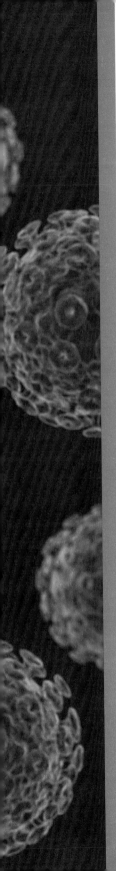

GLOSSARY

AIDS (acquired immunodeficiency syndrome) A late stage of disease caused by the HIV virus in which the immune response is weakened and the person becomes sick from opportunistic infections.

antibody A protein in the blood made by the immune system to fight infection by finding and helping to destroy invading organisms and other substances.

antiretroviral A medication that interferes with replication of retroviruses, such as HIV.

AZT (azidothymidine) The first drug widely used to treat HIV infection.

combination therapy Using more than one antiretroviral drug to treat HIV infection.

condom A latex rubber covering for the penis used to help prevent either pregnancy or the spread of sexually transmitted diseases.

diagnosis The identification of a disease by its signs and symptoms.

DNA (deoxyribonucleic acid) A double-stranded molecule in the nucleus of living cells that contains the genetic information of the organism. Retroviruses, such as HIV, do not have DNA.

epidemic An unexpectedly large number of cases of a disease.

gene A sequence of DNA (or RNA for some viruses, such as HIV) that contains the code to pass a trait from parent to offspring.

genetic material The material within an organism that passes traits from parent to offspring.

hemophilia A disease that prevents the blood from clotting and results in frequent bleeding.

heterosexual A person who is sexually attracted to members of the opposite sex.

HIV (human immunodeficiency virus) A retrovirus that causes AIDS by weakening the immune system.

homophobia A fear of, aversion to, or discrimination against homosexuals.

homosexual A person who is sexually attracted to members of her or his own sex. "Gay" is a term often used to refer to a male homosexual, while "lesbian" refers to a female homosexual.

immune system The body's defense system against disease.

lymph A colorless fluid that circulates throughout the body's tissues.

microorganism An organism too small to be seen with the naked eye, such as a bacterium, fungus, or virus.

monogamy Having only one sex partner.

mutation An accidental change in the DNA or RNA of an organism.

opportunistic infection An infection that occurs because the immune system has been weakened.

replicate To reproduce or make copies.

resistance The ability of an organism to withstand the effects of a drug or antibody that usually would destroy the organism.

retrovirus A virus that has only RNA and must use the cell it infects to produce DNA, RNA, and new viruses. HIV is a retrovirus.

RNA (ribonucleic acid) A single-stranded molecule in the nucleus of living cells that carries information to other parts of the cell and takes part in the making of protein. In some viruses that do not have DNA, such as the retrovirus HIV, RNA contains the virus's genetic information.

vaccine A substance, often injected, that strengthens a person's ability to resist a specific disease.

virus An infectious agent that can replicate only inside another organism's cell, using that cell's machinery.

FOR MORE INFORMATION

Adolescent AIDS Program (AAP)
Children's Hospital at Montefiore Medical Center
111 East 210th Street
Bronx, NY 10467
(718) 882-0232
Web site: http://www.adolescentaids.org
The AAP serves as a local and national resource
    providing information and assistance for those
    living with HIV/AIDS, adolescents at risk, health
    care providers, and families.

AIDSinfo
P.O. Box 6303
Rockville, MD 20849-6303
(800) 448-0440
Web site: http://www.aidsinfo.nih.gov/Other/contact.aspx
    AIDSinfo health information specialists
    provide customized, confidential answers to
    questions about HIV/AIDS clinical trials and
    treatments.

Canadian AIDS Treatment Information
    Exchange (CATIE)
555 Richmond Street West, Suite 381
Box 1104
Toronto, ON M5V 3B1
Canada
(800) 263-1638
Web site: http://www.catie.ca
The CATIE provides information in French and
    English about HIV/AIDS prevention, treatments,
    and new developments.

Centers for Disease Control and Prevention (CDC)

1600 Clifton Road

Atlanta, GA 30333

(800) 232-4636

Web site: http://www.cdc.gov/hiv/contact.htm

The CDC works to improve and protect health by providing
information about risks, new health threats, healthy living
practices, and world health.

Johns Hopkins University School of Medicine

600 N. Wolfe Street

Baltimore, MD 21287

(410) 955-5000

Web site: www.hopkins-aids.edu

Johns Hopkins School of Medicine provides up-to-date
information on the status and developments related to
HIV/AIDS, as well as referrals and other medical
resources.

National Association of People with AIDS (NAPWA)

8401 Colesville Road, Suite 505

Silver Spring, MD 20910

(240) 247-0880

Web site: http://www.napwa.org

The NAPWA is the oldest national AIDS organization as
well as the first network of people living with HIV/AIDS
in the world. It provides HIV/AIDS information and
resources.

Public Health Agency of Canada (PHAV)

130 Colonnade Road

A.L. 6501H

Ottawa, ON K1A 0K9
Canada
Web site: http://www.phac-aspc.gc.ca/index-eng.php
The PHAV provides public health information, resources,
    reports, and records for the citizens of Canada.

Web Sites

Due to the changing nature of Internet links, Rosen
Publishing has developed an online list of Web sites related
to the subject of this book. This site is updated regularly.
Please use this link to access the list:

http://www.rosenlinks.com/epi/aids

FOR FURTHER READING

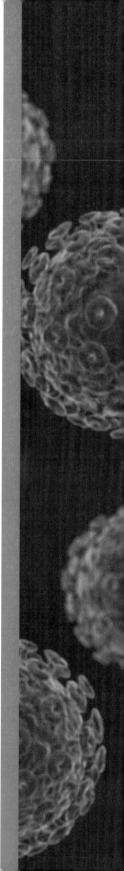

Anonymous. *Quicksand: HIV/AIDS in Our Lives.*
Somerville, MA: Candlewick Press, 2009.

Banish, Roslyn, and Paul A. Volberding. *Focus on
Living: Portraits of Americans with HIV and
AIDS.* Amherst, MA: University of Massachusetts
Press, 2003.

Beck-Sagué, Consuelo, and Caridad Beck. *HIV/AIDS.*
Philadelphia, PA: Chelsea House Publishers, 2004.

Bush, Jenna. *Ana's Story: A Journey of Hope.* New
York, NY: HarperCollins Publishers, 2007.

Critzer, Timothy. *HIV and Me: Firsthand Information
for Coping with HIV and AIDS.* San Francisco, CA:
Firsthand Books, 2004.

D'Adesky, Anne-Christine. *Moving Mountains: The
Race to Treat Global AIDS.* London, England:
Verso, 2004.

Flinn, Alex. *Fade to Black.* New York, NY:
HarperTeen, 2006.

Goldsmith, Connie. *Invisible Invaders: Dangerous
Infectious Diseases.* Minneapolis, MN: Twenty-First
Century Books, 2006.

Howle, Michelle M. *AIDS in the 21st Century: What
You Should Know.* Berkeley Heights, NJ: Enslow
Publishers, Inc., 2003.

Irwin, Alexander, Joyce Millen, and Dorothy Fallows.
*Global AIDS: Myths and Facts, Tools for Fighting
the Aids Pandemic.* Cambridge, MA: South End
Press, 2003.

Minchin, Adele. *The Beat Goes On.* New York, NY:
Simon & Schuster, 2004.

Robinson, Richard. *Frequently Asked Questions About
AIDS and HIV.* New York, NY: Rosen Publishing
Group, 2008.

Stratton, Allan. *Chanda's Secrets*. Toronto, ON, Canada: Annick Press, 2004.

Thomas, Peggy. *Bacteria and Viruses* (Lucent Library of Science and Technology). San Diego, CA: Lucent Books, 2004.

White, Ryan, Anne Marie Cunningham, and Jeanne White. *Ryan White: My Own Story*. New York, NY: New American Library, 1992.

Yount, Lisa, ed. *The Discovery of the AIDS Virus*. San Diego, CA: Greenhaven Press, 2003.

Youth Communication (Organization). *No Excuses: What Teens Can Do to Prevent AIDS* (Quick Insight Series). New York, NY: Youth Communication, 2007.

BIBLIOGRAPHY

Alexander, Ivey L., ed. *AIDS Sourcebook*. 4th ed. Detroit, MI: Omnigraphics, Inc., 2008.

American Psychological Association. "HIV/AIDS and Socioeconomic Status 2009." APA.org. Retrieved September 3, 2009 (http://www.apa.org).

AVERT. "Personal Stories of Men Living with HIV." 2009. Retrieved June 11, 2009. (http://www.avert. org/manstory.htm).

AVERT. "Women, HIV and AIDS." Retrieved June 29, 2000 (http://www.avert.org/women.htm).

AVERT. 'Worldwide HIV and AIDS Statistics." Retrieved June 19, 2009. (http://www.avert.org/ worldwide.htm).

Campbell, Neil A., and Jane B. Reese. *Biology*. 6th ed. Menlo Park, CA: Benjamin Cummings Publishing Company, Inc., 2001.

CDC. "Caregiving in the U.S." April 2004. Retrieved September 6, 2009. (http://www.caregiving.org/ data/04finalreport.pdf).

CDC. "Fact Sheets: HIV/AIDS in the United States." 2008. Retrieved June 13, 2009 (http://www.cdc. gov/hiv/resources/factsheets/us.htm).

CDC. *Morbidity and Mortality Weekly Report*. February 16, 1996. Retrieved June 14, 2009. (http://www.cdc.gov/mmwr/preview/ mmwrhtml/00040227.htm).

CDC. "TB Data and Statistics," June 1, 2009. Retrieved June 22, 2009. (http://www.cdc.gov/tb/ statistics/default.htm).

Ciambrone, Desirée. *Women's Experiences with HIV/ AIDS: Mending Fractured Selves*. New York, NY: Hayworth Press, Inc., 2003.

Clark, Rebecca A., and Robert T. Maupin Jr. *A Woman's Guide to Living with HIV Infection*. Baltimore, MD: John's Hopkins University Press, 2004.

Davidson, Michael W., and Florida State University. "Virus Structure." May 2005. Retrieved June 16, 2009 (http://www. micro.magnet.fsu.edu/cells/virus.html).

Diamond, Jared. "The Mysterious Origin of AIDS." *Natural History*, Vol. 101, No. 9, September 1992, pp. 24–28.

Engel, Jonathan. *The Epidemic: A Global History of AIDS*. New York, NY: Smithsonian Books, 2006.

Goosby, Eric. *Living with HIV/AIDS: The Black Person's Guide to Survival*. Roscoe, IL: Hilton Publishing Company, 2004.

Gross, Jane. "AIDS Patients Face Downside of Living Longer." *New York Times*, January 6, 2008. Retrieved June 9, 2009 (http://nytimes.com/2008/01/06/health/06HIV.html?hp).

Hunter, Susan. *AIDS in America*. New York, NY: Palgrave Macmillan, 2006.

UNAIDS/WHO. "Regional HIV and AIDS Statistics, 2001 and 2007." December 2007. Retrieved June 18, 2009 (http://data.unaids.org/pub/EPI.htm).

UNAIDS/WHO. "2004 Report on the Global AIDS Epidemic." 2004. Retrieved July 23, 2009. (http://unaids. org/bangkok2004/GAR2004_html/ GAR2004_03_en.htm).

UNICEF. *The State of the World's Children 2006: Excluded and Invisible*. New York, NY: United Nations Children's Fund, 2005.

United Nations Information Service. "Coping with HIV/AIDS Within the Family." May 2005. Retrieved June 28, 2009 (http://unis.unvienna.org/unis/pressrels/2005/unisinf73.html).

INDEX

About the Author

Molly Jones is a writer on health and contemporary issues and author of two children's books. She has a Ph.D. in educational research and has done graduate study in epidemiology and biostatistics. Her research has been published in *Medical Care*, *Remedial and Special Education*, and *Journal of Early Intervention*. She lives on Lake Murray near Columbia, South Carolina.

Photo Credits

Front cover (left), back cover (right) © www.istockphoto.com/adisa; front cover (right), back cover (left), pp. 7, 15, 24, 32, 39, 49, 58, 68, 70, 73, 75, 77 © www.istockphoto.com/Felix Mickel; pp. 4–5 Evan Agostini/Getty Images; pp. 8–9, 25 CDC; pp. 10–11 dpphotos/Newscom; pp. 14, 33, 54–55 © AP Images; pp. 16–17 Dr. A. Harrison, Dr. P. Feorino/CDC; p. 19 Kim Stallknecht/AFP/Getty Images; pp. 20–21 © Eye of Science/Photo Researchers, Inc.; pp. 26–27, 50–51 John Chiasson/Getty Images; p. 30 © Véronique Burger/Photo Researchers, Inc.; p. 36 Prakash Singh/AFP/Getty Images; p. 40 James Pozarik/Time & Life Pictures/Getty Images; pp. 42–43 © fine art/Alamy; pp. 44–45 Steve Liss/Time & Life Pictures/Getty Images; p. 46 Chip Somodevilla/Getty Images; pp. 56–57 Luke Frazza/AFP/Getty Images; p. 59 Nicholas Kamm/AFP/Getty Images; p. 61 Terry Ashe/Time & Life Pictures/Getty Images; pp. 62–63 Taro Yamasaki/Time & Life Pictures/Getty Images; pp. 66–67 David McNew/Getty Images

Designer: Sam Zavieh; Editor: Andrea Sclarow; Photo Researcher: Cindy Reiman